THE BOOK OF QUESTIONS

LOVE & SEX

GREGORY STOCK, PH.D.

WORKMAN PUBLISHING, NEW YORK

Copyright © 1989 by Gregory Stock

All rights reserved. No portion of this book may be reproduced—mechanically, electronically, or by any other means, including photocopying—without the written permission of the publisher. Published simultaneously in Canada by Thomas Allen & Son Limited

Library of Congress Cataloging-in-Publication Data
Stock, Gregory.
Love and Sex: the book of questions.
1. Sex customs—Miscellanea. 2. Love—Miscellanea.
3. Interpersonal relations—Miscellanea.
I. Title II. Title: Love and sex.
HQ16.S75 1989
306.7—dc20 89-40371
CIP

ISBN 978-0-89480-619-3

Cover illustration: Tom Lulevitch
Cover design: Charles Kreloff

Workman books are available at special discounts when purchased in bulk for premiums and sales promotions as well as for fund-raising or educational use. Special editions or book excerpts can also be created to specification. For details, contact the Special Sales Director at the address below.

Workman Publishing Company, Inc.
225 Varick Street
New York, NY 10014-4381
www.workman.com

Manufactured in the United States of America

30 29 28

To Angelica,
who melts my heart
and warms my soul.

ACKNOWLEDGMENTS

My special thanks to Lillian McKinstry and Don Ponturo for their thoughtful comments, excellent ideas, and friendly support.

I also thank Melinda Ballou, Lori Campbell, Nick Capasso, Ann Cole, Mary Cunningham, William Jackson, Marina Skumanich, Andrea Southwick, Jane Stock, John Summer, Katherine Turissini, Fred Weber, and Marilyn Zorinado for their assistance and encouragement.

I am grateful to Michael Cader, my editor, for his many excellent suggestions and for his obstinance about a few of them, and to David Breznau for his valuable help with the original THE BOOK OF QUESTIONS.

Finally I thank those friends who, over the years, have told me about their romantic concerns and listened while I talked about mine. Sharing these experiences has expanded my life, taught me a lot about relationships, and deepened and broadened this book enormously.

INTRODUCTION

Love and sex, sex and love—the two are tightly interwoven yet quite separate. They unleash powerful feelings and raise many different questions: What do we really want? What do our feelings mean? The way society treats these matters offers little help. Erotic images surround us, but do they reduce our anxieties about discussing the sexual issues that affect our lives? Ideals of romantic love fill the air, but do they help us handle the everyday realities of a relationship?

Several years ago, while developing THE BOOK OF QUESTIONS, I found that many of the most heartfelt discussions grew from questions about sex and relationships. When I began putting together this book, several friends were enthusiastic about coming up with questions about sex, but uninterested in thinking about issues of love. Wouldn't it sometimes make things easier to be able to separate sexual desire and love? Some people claim to do that, and perhaps they do—at least conceptually. But what I find most interesting—and most confusing—are the tangled ways in which the two interact.

On an intellectual level we may understand that communication is central to a good relationship, but how much do we reveal to loved ones about our inner thoughts and feelings, and how much do we know about theirs? This book can help you explore the challenging issues in your intimate relationships and give you an easy way of bringing up these topics with your friends, family, and lovers. Such discussions can also be fun. After all, these are the subjects that stop us when we are flipping channels on the television. These are the conversations that draw our attention when we overhear them at the next table in a restaurant. And when the discussions are your own, they may help you clarify your values, better understand your needs and desires, and see your friends and partners more clearly.

This is not a test. These are personal questions that have no right or wrong answers—just honest and dishonest ones. They do present you with a decision about openness: How much will you, or should you, reveal about yourself? A big challenge in revealing sensitive personal feelings and information is balancing the need for propriety and privacy against the benefits of candor. You can easily avoid trouble by being very cautious, but you may also miss out on a lot.

When trying to resolve differences with a

partner, it may be tempting to keep little secrets and hope that smoothing over problems will somehow make them disappear. Sometimes this works, but unfortunately the more we avoid difficult issues, the more we wall off parts of our lives—and parts of ourselves—from our loved ones. With too much of that, we may awaken one day to the sad realization that bit-by-bit we have traded away the substance of love for the appearance of it.

Many different issues are included under the theme of "Love and Sex"; some of the questions may touch you deeply, others may seem ridiculous or irrelevant. Your reactions will depend on what issues you happen to be dealing with in your life and can alert you to subjects you should think about more deeply. When you react strongly to a question—even if you hate it—ask yourself why. Are you drawn to questions about sexual exploration? Are you angered by questions about infidelity? Are you bored by questions about falling in love?

As you play with these questions, let yourself be swept up in the situations and dilemmas so that you feel you are really facing them and will have to live with the consequences of your choices. Take them seriously, but don't be afraid to laugh and play. Treat these questions as your own and feel free to tinker with them if it helps make the choices more meaningful to you.

As you listen carefully to what others are saying, you may find that what lies behind someone's answer is even more interesting than the answer itself. Please don't be afraid to use questions of your own to probe responses more deeply and to follow the various tangents that come up. Don't make things too easy for yourself or others, but keep in mind that we all have different levels of comfort with these issues—so be patient. Try to use this book as a tool, not a weapon.

Finally, I hope that in your journey with these questions you will be able to deepen existing friendships and intimacies, form new ones, and gain a greater sense of clarity and joy in your life. Believe in love and give it the honor, trust, and respect it deserves.

*Selected questions are marked with an asterisk to indicate that corresponding follow-up questions can be found at the back of the book, starting on page 189.

THE BOOK OF QUESTIONS

LOVE & SEX

1

If tomorrow you found out that you and your partner had just conceived a child, how would you react? How do you think it might change your relationship?

2

At the beginning of a relationship, do you trust your new partner unless there is something specific to make you do otherwise, or do you withhold your trust until he or she has earned it?

3

When was the last time you made love so spontaneously you couldn't have predicted it 20 minutes before? What attitudes lead to such surprises and what attitudes prevent them from happening?

4

If your lover kept a private journal that was easily accessible, under what circumstances might you read it without permission? For example, what if your relationship were on the rocks and you were confused about your partner's feelings?

5

Would you feel unfaithful if you had frequent sexual daydreams about someone other than your partner? If your partner were having such fantasies, would you want to know about it? Why?

6

Are you more attracted to people whose personalities are similar to yours or very different? What differences attract you and why?

7

Is it important to you to have a particular kind of wedding? If so, under what circumstances would you be willing to forgo that type of ceremony, or even elope?*

8

What implicit agreements between you and your partner are so important that you would leave if they were violated?

9

When did you find out the most about what pleases you sexually and what was it that you learned? Have you discovered more through long-standing relationships or through short periods of intimacy with different lovers?

10

If, during the next month, you could have the power to hear your partner's every thought when you made love, would you want to? Would it upset you to have your partner hear your thoughts?

11

Have you ever felt that your involvement with your partner was more hard work than fun? If so, do you feel this is to be expected or is a sign that something basic is wrong?

12

When you meet people do you ever imagine what they would look like naked or what they are like sexually? How would you feel if you knew someone were musing about you in this way?

13

In what ways do you and your partner compete with each other?

14

If starting now you could have $500 a day until you next touched your lover, how long do you think you would avoid physical contact? How do you think this unusual offer would affect your relationship?

15

If you were sick and feeling miserable, would you rather be by yourself or have your partner with you? Why?

16

Are there any erotic pleasures you once looked at as "weird" or disgusting but now relish? Would you like to try new things with your partner more or less than you do now?*

17

If during a two-week vacation you had met and fallen in love with someone who lived a thousand miles from you, what would you do when you returned home to give the relationship a chance? If the two of you wanted to be together, how would you be willing to change your life to make it happen, and how much would you expect your lover to change?

18

Where is the most unusual place you ever had sex? Is there any illicit or dangerous place you've thought would be fun to try if you had the chance? If so, what appeals to you about it?

19

Have you remained close friends with any former lovers? If not, would you like to have done so?

20

When you first have sex with someone, is it more important to you that your partner is a "good" lover or that your partner thinks you are a "good" lover?

21

If you were dating several people and one sent you a love note and flowers, would you hide them or display them openly? If you displayed the flowers and one of the others asked about them, what would you say?

22

MEN: Have you ever had a traumatic experience as a result of being unable to get an erection? If so, what was your biggest concern at the time and how would you have liked your partner to behave?

WOMEN: Have you ever had an unpleasant lovemaking experience because your partner could not get an erection? If so, what went through your mind when you first suspected this was going to happen and what was the worst thing about the experience? How would you have liked your partner to behave?

23

Are you more inclined to threaten, cajole, reason, or plead when trying to get your way? When none of this works and you and your partner can't agree about something important, what do you do?

24

If you and your lover were in a hotel room with a squeaky bed and walls so thin that you could hear voices in the next room, how much would it affect your lovemaking? What if you faced the same conditions at a friend's house?

25

Are heart-to-heart talks more often a way for you and your partner to share feelings or to solve problems? Is that how you want it to be?

26

If you caught a long-term relationship virus (LTRV) that would kill you if you stayed in a romantic involvement for more than six months, how do you think your partners would differ from those you now like? Do you think you would end up spending more or less energy on sex and romance?

27

If as a result of an injury or illness you could never again have intercourse, do you think your lover would adjust to the change or eventually leave you because of it? How would you adjust to it?*

28

If you were single, what rules would you have about seeing people who were already involved with someone or who had just broken up? What about co-workers or other people you deal with on a daily basis? What experiences have led you to these rules?

29

If you lost your eyesight, in what ways do you think your notions of a perfect partner would change?

30

Would it upset you to see a good friend or sibling become seriously involved with a former lover of yours? If so, why do you think you would feel this way? What is the longest you remember having felt possessive about an ex-lover?

31

What little romantic attentions would please your lover most? How long has it been since you last paid them, and why don't you do so more frequently?

32

If you inherited $100,000, would you expect to have more say than your spouse about how it was used? What if your spouse inherited the money?*

33

If you wanted to have sex and your partner didn't, would you rather have your partner rebuff your advances or go through the motions for your benefit?*

34

How long do you think you could tolerate spending virtually every minute of every day with your partner? Assume you would work together, eat together, play together, and sleep together. Which one of you needs more time apart?

35

If you learned that a 50-year-old woman was engaged to be married to a man of 21, what would your first reaction be? How would you feel differently if the ages were reversed so that the woman was 21 and the man 50?*

36

Would you rather have a strikingly attractive spouse who was disappointing in bed, or a plain-looking one who was fantastic in bed?

37

When you have sex with someone for the first time, do you feel you are making an implicit commitment even if nothing is stated? If so, what is that commitment, and how does it change if your intimacy continues for a number of weeks or months?*

38

If today you had to decide irrevocably whether you would marry and spend the rest of your life with your partner, or separate and never see each other again, which would you choose and why? Assume that all prior promises and commitments are set aside and that there are no children involved.

39

When you fall in love, do you get so caught up that you almost lose contact with your friends? If so, do you think this upsets them?*

40

If your partner completely lost his or her temper and started smashing dishes and furniture, what would you do? What would you do if the anger were directed at you and you were slapped, hit, or threatened? What would you do if either of these started happening every six months or so?

41

If you began to be bored when you were with your partner, would you start trying to find new ways you could enjoy being together, or would you start developing more ways of enjoying yourself independently? Would you discuss this problem with your partner or try to hide it?

42

When was the last time you felt so in love you were almost overwhelmed by your emotions? If you didn't tell your lover how strongly you were touched, why didn't you?

43

In a romantic context, have you ever pretended to care about someone much more than you really did? If so, did you do it to make someone else jealous, to try to get something from the person, or for some other reason?

44

If drugs or alcohol dramatically enhanced you and your partner's pleasure in sex, would you want to use them regularly?

45

Do you find particular environmental undercurrents especially stimulating sexually—for example, danger, opulence, or formality? If so, do you ever try to create situations that contain these elements? What is the most sensuous, erotic setting you can imagine for lovemaking?

46

What kinds of problems in a relationship are better smoothed over to maintain a friendly tone, and what kinds are better confronted openly no matter how threatening that prospect seems?

47

In what ways do you experience and express your love differently from the way your partner does? Do such differences ever lead you to feel that one of you loves more deeply than the other?

48

What do you think it would be like to spend a few days with your lover and not communicate verbally?

49

If you and a close friend were attracted to each other and neither of you were involved with anyone else, do you think you would be jeopardizing your friendship if you decided to have sex?

50

WOMEN: You have serious medical complications midway into your first pregnancy and without an abortion there is a 25 percent chance that neither you nor your baby will survive. Knowing you will never again be able to become pregnant, would you have an abortion? Would you give much weight to your husband's feelings in the matter?

MEN: Under the above circumstances, would you urge your wife to have the child or to have an abortion? How would you feel if she decided upon the other alternative?

51

If you could send your partner to a sexual-techniques school, would you? Assume your lover would come home an expert after spending three months studying and practicing the art of lovemaking.*

52

Do you think you or your partner has discussed more openly with confidants the details of your sex life and your relationship?*

53

If you were involved with someone and started toying with the idea of marriage, would you hesitate to mention this until you were fairly certain of your feelings? What do you think would be the biggest risk of bringing up the subject before then?

54

In what ways, if any, do you use your sexuality to get special treatment from other people? In what ways—either consciously or unconsciously—do your friends or your partners do this?

55

Has your parents' relationship influenced you more as a healthy model to imitate or an unhealthy one to avoid?*

56

Have you ever been in love not so much with the person you were seeing but rather with your image of that person and the life the two of you could have together? If so, were you aware of this at the time?

57

If your 15-year-old daughter were raped and became pregnant, would you want her to have an abortion? What if she got pregnant after getting drunk at a party and ending up having sex with a boy she hardly knew?

58

How much do marriage vows actually mean to you?

59

If you went out with someone a few times and you both were attracted to each other, do you think you could stimulate the person's interest in you more by having sex or by withholding sex?

Do you find shy people more sexually attractive than outgoing people or less so? How do you respond to other personality types?

61

When someone you like has much stronger feelings for you than you can reciprocate, do you push them away for their own good, tell them how you feel and let them decide what to do, ignore the matter and enjoy yourself, or something else? If roles were reversed, what would you like the other person to do?

62

How did you find out how to have sex? Can you think of a better way to have picked this up? How would you like your kids to learn about sex?

63

Roughly how many times do sexual thoughts come into your mind in an average day?

64

What do you do to try to hold on to your partner's love? Would you find it more painful to have your partner stop loving you, leave you, or die in an auto accident?*

65

Assume that the only birth control method is a pill that can be taken by either men or women and is 100 percent effective. One pill lasts for two years and has just one side effect: it causes a bad headache every other week. Would you offer to take the first pill if you and your spouse decided to use them?

66

What one thing do you think would most draw the opposite sex to you: better looks, more education, more money, more confidence, or something else?

67

Would you rather suffer a nerve injury that numbed your entire genital region, or one that made you completely deaf?

68

Are there times you feel your partner is someone you don't really know? What aspects of your partner's personality or background do you least understand, and how much do you care about understanding these things?*

69

How many times in your life have you felt more in love than ever before? How many times have you been with someone you felt you would be with forever?

70

If you were confident that their choice would be a good one, would you be willing to have your parents select your spouse? If not, why not?

71

Have your most enduring relationships been those in which you knew your partner for a long time or only a short time before having sex? What do you consider a "long" or "short" time?

72

Have you ever had sexual thoughts about members of your own family? If so, how did you handle those feelings?

73

Have you ever talked with people much older than you about how their experience of sex has changed over the years? If not, is it because you aren't interested or because you feel awkward about bringing up the topic?

74

When was the last time you were willing to hurt your lover by telling a painful truth you felt he or she needed to hear?*

75

Do you find emotional or physical pain more difficult to handle? For example, would you suffer more by going through life afflicted with severe, recurring migraines, or by having your heart broken again and again?

76

Do you think your friends believe your sex life is better or worse than it actually is?

77

What in someone's life—for instance, religion, occupation, ethnic background, age, health, or marital history—would keep you from marrying a person you had somehow already fallen in love with?*

78

When you look back on past romances, do you ever wonder what you saw in a former lover? If so, is it more because you have changed or because you have grown to see the person more clearly?

79

What words do you use for different sex acts and sexual parts of the body, and in what situations might you use them? For example, what different nuances do "make love," "sleep together," "spend the night with someone," and "have sex" have for you?

80

If you had to spend one month each year separated from your spouse and kids, what sorts of things might you do during the period? Do you think your relationship would be strengthened or weakened by recurring separations of this sort?

81

How do you react when someone "gives you the eye" in a public place? In what situations do you flirt, and why do you do it?

82

If you did something thoughtless, would you rather your lover became loudly angry for a few hours or quietly annoyed for a few days? When your lover is angry with you and won't admit it, how do you know and what do you do?

83

Have you ever had a lover you wanted to break up with but keep as a friend? or perhaps as a casual sexual partner?

84

If a month before your wedding your wealthy fiancé(e) suggested drawing up a prenuptial agreement specifying the financial terms of any divorce, how would you react? What kind of terms do you think would be fair in such an agreement?

85

If you were certain you would neither catch any diseases nor suffer any social consequences from your behavior, would you ever be willing to pay someone to have sex with you?*

86

If your partner greatly enjoyed some activity that held no interest for you, would you be more likely to try to become interested in it, encourage your partner to do it without you, discourage the activity, or handle it some other way? Why?

87

If one day you were to learn that several years earlier your spouse had deceived you by having a brief affair, how do you think it would change your relationship?

88

What is the most planning and energy you have ever put into a romantic event? Was the planning worth it, or might everything have gone as well without it?

89

Would you rather your lover had a beautiful face and an average body, or an average face and a beautiful body?

90

If after medical checkups you found you tested negative for exposure to AIDS and your partner tested positive, what would you do? Assume that the exposure was probably from a blood transfusion.

91

In selecting a life partner, do you think it is more important to follow your heart or your head? Would you ever let yourself fall in love with someone who wasn't at all like the image of the person you would hope to find?

92

Who initiates sex more often, you or your partner? When one of you feels like having sex, how does he or she let the other know? Ideally, how would you like your partner to go about initiating sex?

93

What was the worst heartbreak you ever suffered? How did it affect your feelings about intimacy and love? All things considered, do you feel the experience was good or bad for you?*

94

Do you feel that your responsibilities to your partner keep you from doing the things you really want to do? Have you ever used such responsibilities as an excuse for avoiding things you were afraid of?

95

Thinking of all the ways that your partner differs from you as a person, what one difference do you treasure the most?

96

What would you do if you discovered that your 12-year-old son had been playing sexual games with your neighbor's 6-year-old daughter? What if the young girl were yours and the boy, your neighbor's?

97

How much energy do you put into sex and romance when you are first getting to know someone, and how much do you put in after you are involved in a long-term relationship? Does your enjoyment of sex and romance depend more upon how much energy you devote to it, or upon how long you've known someone?

98

Are there times you would rather masturbate than have sex with a partner? If so, when?

99

Five years from now, in what ways do you think your relationship will have improved or deteriorated?

100

Could you fall in love with someone you weren't attracted to sexually?*

101

Does the thought of physical force during sex excite you in any way?

102

If you were exposed to a poison that permanently blocked your ability to experience orgasm yet in no way altered your sensory feelings, how do you think it would change your sex life? What if your partner were exposed to this chemical rather than you?

103

What is the longest lovemaking experience you've ever had?

104

MEN: If you and your wife wanted children but you discovered you were sterile, would you want to forgo children, adopt a child, or have your wife become pregnant through artificial insemination with donor sperm? Which do you think your wife would want?

WOMEN: If you and your husband wanted children but you found you were infertile, would you want to forgo children, adopt a child, or have your husband impregnate another woman who agreed to bear the child for you? Which do you think your husband would want?

105

When you start getting seriously involved with someone, do you want the person to stop going out with others? How deeply involved would you let yourself become before insisting upon this sort of commitment?

106

In what joint activities do you support and help your partner while he or she runs the show, and in what activities does your partner do this for you?

107

If you could have Cupid shoot a magic arrow that would make any one person you chose love and adore you forever, would you? If so, whom would you pick?

108

Do you think saying "I love you" to someone means more or less to you than it does to other people? What about having sex?

109

If all your responsibilities were suspended while you and your lover took a one-month, all-expense-paid vacation to the place of your choice, where would you go? Would you choose some other place if you were taking the vacation by yourself?

110

Where do you and your lover find it easiest to have intimate and heartfelt talks? How good are you about not bringing up important topics at the wrong time or place?

111

Are you willing to change your appearance to make yourself more attractive to your partner, or do you feel your partner should love you just the way you are? For example, how much are you willing to modify your hairstyle or change the way you dress?

112

Have you ever spied on a lover you didn't trust? If so, what provoked your behavior and did you ever admit what you had done?

113

Do you reach a more intense orgasm through intercourse, oral sex, masturbation, or having your partner touch you? If you had to permanently give up two of these, which would you choose?

114

If you were to die today in an accident, how long would you want your partner to wait before moving on and finding someone new? Why? If your partner died, how long do you think it would be before you recovered enough to be capable of loving again?

115

What is the most selfless, caring thing you can remember having done for someone? Were you in love with that person?*

116

Why do you think so many single people wish they were married and so many married people wish they were single? Do you think many of these people would be happier if they were granted their wishes?

117

If your partner of many years were going through a period of personal crisis and wanted to live alone for six months to figure things out, might you agree or would such an arrangement be unthinkable and signify the end of your relationship?

118

When and where did you lose your virginity? Since then, what has been the longest time you've ever gone without sex?

119

Would you rather have a mate twice as bright as you or half as bright? What about twice as attractive? Why?

120

Assume you are to be blessed with one lover you adore and one soul mate you can talk to about anything. Would you rather have these be two separate individuals or one and the same person? Why?

121

How much of your enjoyment of sex comes from giving pleasure to your partner? Could you enjoy yourself if you knew your partner took little pleasure in the experience?

122

Will you ever be too old to fall head-over-heels in love? If so, when and why?*

123

If you became extremely frustrated and unhappy with your spouse, would you be more likely to leave or have an affair? How bad would things have to get before you would consider such an action?*

124

Have you ever felt jealous of the warmth and attention a partner has given to a pet or child? If so, do you think he or she knew how you were feeling?

125

Would you like to see intimate journals and letters your lover wrote during a previous romance that took place long before you knew each other? If so, why?

126

What is the best thing you have discovered about your partner since you became involved with each other? In what ways have you grown to respect your partner more as time has passed?

127

If your partner were accused of a serious crime and subjected to a long and humiliating public trial, how loyal and supportive would you be?

128

What are the main things you feel you want or need from a life partner? How are these different from what they were when you first began to think about such things?

129

Do you think you would ever enjoy having your lover pretend to be someone else during lovemaking? If so, what "make-believe" role might appeal to you? Would you be willing to pretend to be another person if it would excite your lover?

130

Would you rather your lover were more jealous or less jealous of you? What could you do to bring this about?

131

Would you rather have everyone envy you because they admire and like your partner, who is actually not such a great catch; or have everyone shake their heads and think you could have done better, yet know yourself that your partner is actually wonderful?

132

Could you be happy spending only half of each year with your mate? If you had to have such a relationship, in what size chunks would you want to take your time together?

133

Given the current state of contraceptives, do you think you or your partner should be responsible for birth control?

134

In what ways do you feel that you and your partner have a stronger relationship than other couples you know have?

135

If you could have one night of sex with anyone in the world you desired—but only if you got a note of permission from your partner—would you ask for it?

136

MEN: In dating, do you prefer to pay for everything or only for yourself? How do your expectations change when you pay? What about when your date pays for both of you?

WOMEN: In dating, do you prefer to pay your own way or be treated? How does paying for yourself change your attitude about the evening? Do you ever pay for your date, and if so, how do you feel about it?

137

If your lover left you for someone else, would you find it more painful if your rival were a man or a woman? Why?

138

If you could be twice as passionately in love with your partner as you are now, would you want to be? What about 10 times as in love? At what point is love so strong it is unhealthy?

139

At your age, do you think it is easier for men or for women to find a good partner? In what ways do you think the aging process is different for men and women?*

140

When and where do you make love most often? If you could vary either the time or the place more than you do now, which would you prefer?

141

What is your biggest fear about making a total commitment to someone? What does being totally committed mean to you?

142

What couple has the best relationship you've seen? What about their relationship most appeals to you?

143

What does your partner do that makes you feel most loved? Do you think your partner is aware of this?

144

What is the oldest a person could be whom you could find sexually stimulating? What is the youngest? How would you have answered when you were half your age, and how do you think you will answer in 20 years?

145

If you and your partner were having frequent arguments and problems, and your partner wanted the two of you to start seeing a therapist, would you be willing to do so? If not, why not?

146

If a perfect contraceptive were developed and all venereal disease disappeared, how would you change your sexual behavior?

147

What one change in your behavior would be most likely to make your relationship with your partner closer and warmer? Why don't you make that change?

148

In past romantic breakups, have you or your former partners suffered more? When a romance fails, do you think it is better to sever contact or to continue to communicate while you are separating?*

149

When was the last time you got angry or frustrated about things outside your relationship and then vented those feelings on your partner? How do you react when your partner says you are doing this?

150

Under what circumstances might you pretend you were enjoying sex much more than you actually were?

151

How much of falling in love is illusion and how much is real chemistry?

152

If you came into great wealth, would you be afraid of being taken for a ride by someone who was after you for your money? How would you protect yourself without being overly suspicious of people?

153

If your 9-year-old son told you that his 12-year-old sister was planning to have sex with her boyfriend, what would you do?

154

If you and your partner began to have sexual problems, would you look for underlying causes or try to figure out some direct way of improving your lovemaking?*

155

How long would you be willing to support a spouse who was going to school? recuperating from an illness? writing novels that weren't published?

156

What is the strongest public display of affection you ever made? What is the strongest one you ever witnessed, and how did you react to it? At what point do you think expressing affection in public becomes improper?

157

What is the most romantic thing you have ever done or had done for you?

158

How has the role that sex plays in your life changed over the years? Are you comfortable with this change?*

159

One night, after going out for a few drinks with some old friends visiting town, your spouse comes home pale and shaken and tells you of having just run over a child who darted into the street. After stopping and discovering that the child was dead, your mate realized that no one else had seen the accident, and then fled. Knowing that confessing to the crime would lead to several years of imprisonment, and that keeping quiet about it would always keep the secret between the two of you, what would you want your spouse to do? How strongly would you insist on that course of action?*

160

How do you feel when your partner tells you that you don't listen enough or don't express yourself enough? What about when your partner dismisses what you say as being illogical or not making sense?

161

Would you want to live with a prospective mate before getting married? If so, for about how long?

162

If every day next year you had an extra hour of leisure, would you rather spend all of it with your partner or by yourself? Assumc it must be one or the other.

163

If you could watch a video of yourself making love, would you want to?

164

When you are attracted to someone and another person begins to show a lot of interest in him or her, does it strengthen or diminish your own feelings? Has such a competitive urge ever led you to believe you were more in love with someone than you really were?*

165

How much do you treasure the memories you have of the special moments you and your partner have shared together? How would your feelings for your partner be different if you had no such precious memories to recall?

166

What type of body do you respond to most strongly? Who comes to mind when you try to think of someone sexy you've seen recently?*

167

If for some reason you could never again be sexually intimate with anyone of the opposite sex, would you seek such intimacy with someone of your own sex? To begin to seem sexually appealing to you, what would someone of your own sex have to be like?

168

In what ways are you able to love someone more deeply now than when you were younger? How did this change come about?

169

You are beginning an exciting romance and learn that your partner, who badly wants children, would almost certainly leave you if he or she discovered that you were unable to have kids. If you were almost sure that you could never have a child, would you try to hide the fact for a while or reveal it right away?

170

If your lover died and you could keep only one thing to remember him or her by, what would you want? If you were dying and could leave only one of your possessions to your mate, what would it be?

171

How frequently do you give your partner your full and undivided attention and try to understand exactly what he or she is saying and feeling?

172

Do you consider yourself sexually adventurous? What experiences lead you to view yourself in this way?

173

If you could either double or halve your desire for sex, which would you do? How do you think such a change would alter your relationship?

174

Assume you are happily married to a partner you are not passionate about but love dearly. If you chanced upon someone who made you feel better than you had ever felt before, and who you knew was equally in love with you, what would you do?

175

Do you seek advice about romantic issues more or less than about other things in your life?*

176

Have you ever been in love with someone you knew you could not trust? If you found yourself in such a dangerous involvement, would you try to leave?

177

If you met someone and really wanted the person to be attracted to you, what would you do to help that happen?

178

When does sex make you feel guilty? Has this changed as you have grown older?

179

If you had to choose something new for your partner to do to you when you make love, what would you pick? Is there anything that used to excite you a lot but that now excites you much less than your lover thinks it does?*

180

In what ways do you try to change yourself to please your partner?

181

Have you ever loved deeply enough to be willing to sacrifice your own life to save your lover? If so, when in your relationship did your feelings reach that point? If not, do you think you will ever feel that strongly?

182

On your 25th anniversary, what kind of honeymoon do you think would be most pleasing to look back upon?*

183

If you and your spouse had a passionate, intoxicating love you knew would last only until the day a child was born, would you have a child? Assume that after your child's birth your relationship would still be warm and affectionate but not passionate.

184

How much of your week would you like to spend having sex if you had a willing partner and enough time?

185

If you and the partner of an acquaintance were very attracted to each other, and you knew that the two of them were having a lot of problems, what would you do? Assume you are single.*

186

Would you prefer a wild, passionate, turbulent relationship or a calm, warm, consistent one? Why?

187

Imagine that your sister-in-law worked as a waitress for seven years to put your brother through college and law school, and that for the last four years she has been a housewife and mother supported by his excellent salary. If he wanted a divorce and asked for your honest advice, how would you suggest treating his future salary in the settlement?

188

The last time you were really mad at your partner, did you express it openly or try to hide it? Would it be better for your relationship if you expressed your anger more or hid it more?

189

Can sex that is predictable excite you, or must there be a touch of the unexpected to keep you stimulated?

190

If your partner went out of town to a friend's wedding and after a wild reception ended up having sex with an old flame, would you want to be told? Assume that the two of them had a great time but planned no further contact, and that no one else was aware of what had happened. How do you think such an admission would affect your relationship? If the situation were reversed, would you say anything to your partner?

191

Do you tend to fall in love with someone more because of the dynamic between you as a couple, or because of who that person is as an individual?

192

If you found out that some young kids with binoculars had watched through your window while you made love, how would you react? If you were hiking in the woods and came across two teenagers making love in a field, would you keep still and watch?

193

Do you get a deeper pleasure from loving or from being loved?

194

Would you rather have a wonderful and enduring marriage after painful growth in two previous broken marriages, or have a decent first marriage that lasts?

195

Do you have any sexual fantasies that you hide from your lover because they seem too personal or too dangerous to share with anyone? If so, what do you think would happen if you revealed them?

196

How many times have you fallen in love and allowed yourself to just be swept away? How many times have you felt yourself falling in love and blocked the feeling because you were afraid of what could happen?

197

Have you ever answered or written a personals ad? If so, are you glad you did it? If not, have you ever toyed with the idea?

198

If you and your partner were to separate, would it hurt more to lose your hopes for the future or the daily companionship you now share?

199

When was the last time you had so much fun making love that you laughed out loud? Are your fondest memories of lovemaking from times that were playful or serious?

200

Would you find it more distressing to never have kids or to never have an enduring marriage?*

201

If you could resculpt any part of your body with free, safe, cosmetic surgery, would you? How do you think doing so would change your life?

202

Would you ever marry someone over the strong opposition of your entire family?

203

Does your partner do things that regularly embarrass you? If so, how do you handle this?

204

If a close friend reported seeing your partner having a very romantic dinner with someone, but your partner absolutely denied being there, whom would you tend to believe? How strong would the evidence have to be before you'd accept that your spouse was lying to you?

205

What is the most unpleasant sexual experience you can recall? In what ways do you think this experience has had a positive influence on your life? a negative influence?

206

Can you think of times you felt in love with someone and later realized you weren't? If so, what led you to see things more clearly and what did you decide had actually been going on?*

207

Most people play games in their relationships, yet most people claim they don't. What games do you now play, and what games that you used to play have you given up?

208

How would you rate yourself as a lover? In what ways do you think you could improve?*

209

If you had a terrific sexual and emotional relationship with your partner, would you be more disturbed to learn that your partner occasionally had brief sexual flings, or regularly had sexual fantasies about other people? Why?

210

Your closest friend (and companion since childhood) and your lover (whom you have known only three months but feel like you have waited for all your life) are both in grave danger. If you could save only one, which would it be?

211

Do you and your partner still have the same roles and expectations that you fell into when you were first getting to know each other? If so, in what ways would you now like to change them, and how would your partner feel about that?

212

How promiscuous would you be if you knew your mate would be as faithful as you wished and, without resentment, give you any sexual freedoms you asked for?

213

Do you generally become more or less sexually attracted to a lover as you become increasingly familiar and at ease with each other? Why do you think this is so and what do you think it reveals about you?

214

After ending a relationship and sticking with that decision for a while, have you ever changed your mind and gone back to the person? If so, why did you do it and how was it different the second time around?

215

Do you think it would be possible for a talented actor or actress to capture your heart by doing and saying all of the "right" things? If so, what behavior would be most likely to succeed with you?

216

If your next child would be an exact genetic clone of either yourself or your spouse, which would you prefer? Why?*

217

Some say that love is blind. Are there any big differences in the way you and other people view your partner? If so, why do you think other people miss what seems so clear to you and vice versa?

218

If you had a fixed amount of time, energy, and love to give to those you care about, what fraction would you give to your lover? How would you divide what remains among the other people in your life?

219

Have you ever loved someone you didn't respect? If so, did it make you respect yourself any less?

220

If you had been seeing someone for a few weeks and you both were very attracted to each other, do you think you would be more likely to eventually get married if you started sleeping together or if you resisted doing so? If you wanted to have sex and the other person refused, how long would it take for you to consider ending the romance?

221

What is the most open discussion of sex you have had with your parents? What about with your brothers or sisters?

222

While you and your spouse are vacationing overseas, you meet a friendly wealthy couple at your hotel and have dinner with them. That evening, when your spouse goes to the rest room, they politely offer you $50,000 in cash if you both will join them for a one-night sexual orgy. How would you reply? Would you discuss their proposition with your spouse?

223

What is the greatest number of sexual partners you have had in one week? in one year?

224

In what ways would you like to have a greater sense of either togetherness or independence in your relationship? How do you think your partner feels about this?

225

Upon meeting the love of your life, would you rather be a virgin and discover your sexuality within the relationship, or already possess extensive sexual experience to share with your partner? Similarly, would you want your mate to be sexually experienced already? Regardless of your current situation, assume that the choice is yours to make now.

226

In the early phases of a romance, how much are you influenced by your friends' and family's opinions of your potential partner?

227

If you were to give advice to someone a few years younger than you about the best way to find a mate, what would you recommend?

228

If your partner were gone for two months, what things that he or she takes care of would be a real problem for you?*

229

Would you be willing to donate sperm for artificial insemination (or eggs for embryo implantation) to help infertile couples have children? If so, would knowing you had children you knew nothing about be pleasing or disturbing to you? How would you feel about your spouse doing this?

230

Have you ever been in love with someone and yet never told the person how you felt? If so, why?

231

Would you rather be passionate about the mate you choose but have few interests or beliefs in common, or feel little passion but share many common interests and beliefs?

232

You and your spouse have been unsuccessfully struggling to have a child for some time and today is the day—one of the year's 12 peak days for conception. If the two of you were having a nasty fight, would you still go ahead and have sex?

233

People often proclaim that marriage is "for better or for worse." What in your present relationship has proved to be better than you imagined when you first met? What has been worse? How do you think your partner would reply to the same question?

234

What do you think makes someone a great lover? What fraction of what you own would you be willing to give up in order to be one of the best lovers in the world?

235

When did you first realize your parents had sex? How frequently do you think they have sex now? Have you ever had sex in your parents' house?*

236

Was there any period in your life when you were particularly stimulated by pornography? If so, why do you think you were drawn to it and how did it affect you?

237

If you and your lover knew everything about each other, how do you think your relationship would be different? What things, if any, are better kept private in a relationship?

238

If your partner had a fabulous, once-in-a-lifetime career opportunity, but would have to go to a distant country and be separated from you for two years to take advantage of it, would you be in favor of it? If your partner went, would you be faithful and expect the same?

239

What is the best lovemaking experience you remember? What made it so special for you?

240

Can you recall any sexual or erotic experiences you had as a child? If so, how do you think these experiences continue to affect your life today?

241

If your partner had a fatal heart attack tonight, what would you most regret not having done together? When do you think you will actually get around to doing those things?

242

If you had to make love either in total darkness or where background noise would prevent speech, which would you prefer? Why?

243

What are the most significant milestones for you in the evolution of an intimate, committed relationship? For example, in what ways do your expectations change when you first kiss and hold someone? first say you love someone? start seeing someone exclusively? or first mention marriage?

FURTHER QUESTIONS

Just as our responses to these questions are highly personal, so are our interpretations of them. One person may feel that a question deals with loyalty and trust; another person may feel the same question looks at sexual desire; and a third may feel it concerns communication.

The purpose of these further questions is not to tell you what the important issues are in this book; that is up to you. They are here to extend some ideas posed in the earlier questions and to invite you to do likewise with the questions you find intriguing.

Most of the value of these questions will come from actively exploring them. Good personal questions do not lead to an answer as much as they lead to more questions.

7

How important is ceremony to you? Could you feel as deeply bonded to someone without a marriage ceremony? If you felt no pressure from any family or friends, what kind of wedding would you have?

16

If your lover asked you to do something sexual that you found distasteful, would you try to overcome your feelings or simply refuse?

27

Following your incapacitation, would you rather have your lover try to do without sex, search with you for new ways of being satisfied, or look elsewhere for sex? Would any of these approaches be unacceptable to you? What would you want to do if roles were reversed?

32

In your marriage, what money or other possessions, if any, do you believe should be entirely yours and not jointly owned by you and your spouse? If you were involved with someone for many years—but not married—how would you like to handle money and expenses?

33

How do you feel and behave when your partner isn't responsive to your overtures for sex or tenderness? When roles are reversed and you aren't in the mood for sex, will you usually oblige your partner or not? What do you think would happen if you had sex only when you really wanted to?

35

Would your reaction be different if instead of planning a marriage, the two—separated in age by 30 years—were simply having an affair? What do you think would be the best thing about being romantically involved with someone significantly older or younger?

37

If your expectations about a relationship change significantly after you first have sex, do you discuss this before you have sex, afterwards, or not at all? Have your partners generally shared your attitudes about commitment or have they had quite different ideas?

39

How do you feel when a friend falls in love and no longer seems to have any time for you? Do you know any people who appear to use their friends and acquaintances mostly to fill in the gaps between romantic involvements? Do you think that focusing all of one's attention on a lover at the beginning of a relationship fosters an unhealthy dependence on that person, or is it simply a healthy part of being in love?

51

Beyond fairly elementary skills, how much do you think sexual technique contributes to the overall quality of lovemaking? How much knowledge about sexual techniques is sufficient for you? Do you think it is closer to the truth to say that a good lover is someone who is skilled in sexual techniques, or someone who is able to develop a strong rapport with his or her partner?

52

In general, do you think men or women talk more freely about their sex lives and their romances? Why do you think this is so? Are there things about your relationship that you might talk about with someone else, but nevertheless would expect your partner not to reveal to anyone? Do you care whether other people view you as a good partner or not?

55

Are there ways in which your parents treat each other that you do not like, but somehow—despite your efforts to do otherwise—seem to have imitated in your own involvements? If so, do you have any idea why you have been unable to break these patterns?

64

Do you think that losing your lover would hurt you more or less than others might guess from the way the two of you behave together and speak about each other? What are the everyday things in your relationship you would miss the most if your partner were no longer a part of your life?

68

Do you ever feel resentful because your partner doesn't understand you better? What do you do to help your partner understand those parts of you that he or she least comprehends?

74

After your immediate distress passes, do you generally feel more resentment or gratitude toward someone who has told you an unpleasant truth about yourself? When you tell a person something you know he or she will have difficulty hearing, do you think beforehand about how best to get the person to be open to what you have to say?

77

What character and personality traits are so important that you would never marry someone who you felt lacked them?

85

Do you feel that prostitution should be illegal? If so, why? Can you discern any elements of prostitution in more accepted romantic interactions? If so, what are they?

93

Do you think it is possible to experience love without also suffering feelings of pain and loss?

100

Have you ever confused sexual attraction and love? To what extent can you separate physical attraction and emotional love? What would you do if, as a result of a permanent change in his or her appearance, you no longer felt physically attracted to your mate?

115

When you are in love with someone, do you generally behave in a loving fashion? What does it mean to be "loving" to someone? If someone loves you and yet doesn't treat you with love, do you still value their love? If so, why?

122

Can a person know too much about life to be able to fall in love? How much of the power of falling in love comes from the wonder of experiencing emotions for the first time? Are you capable of feeling as much love and passion now as you did when you were younger?

123

At what periods in your life have you been most vulnerable to the temptations of an affair? What was it you were seeking from another person at those times? Have you ever seriously contemplated and then consciously avoided an affair? If so, what stopped you?

139

How well do you feel you understand the opposite sex? Which sex do you think has the most difficult role in dating? in marriage? in lovemaking? in going through puberty? What makes you feel this is so?

148

If you left someone you had been seeing for several years, would you feel a responsibility to help your former lover get over you? If you would, and if you soon became involved with someone new, do you think you would still devote time and energy to helping your ex-partner? If the shoe were on the other foot, how much help would you expect from your former lover?

154

What do you feel are the best indicators that problems are brewing in a relationship? Do you think that the quality of sex you are having with your partner can serve as a reliable barometer to warn you of relationship storms approaching on the horizon?

158

Is sex more a way for you to express your love or to gratify your physical needs? How might it be good for you to have a lover who used sex in the other way?

159

At what point might personal or family concerns lead you to override your feelings of right and wrong? How harshly would you judge someone who hid a serious crime out of concern for his or her spouse or child? If you were the spouse of the hit-and-run driver in the incident described, and the judge instructed you to determine the punishment for your mate, what would you come up with?

164

If you were strongly drawn to someone, would your interest be fueled more if you saw that the person was very attracted to you, or if you saw that the person had little interest in you?

166

Do you feel that it is all right to have sex without being in love? What feelings must you have before sex with someone feels right to you? How deeply involved can you be with a person if the mutual attraction between you is almost entirely sexual?

175

When you are in love, is outside opinion worth less because your feelings are so personal, or worth more because it is so easy for you to lose perspective? How much do you trust your insights about what is best for someone else?

179

Do you communicate the simple things you want during sex or do you expect your partner to somehow figure out what you like? If you don't, is it more because you are unsure of what pleases you, or because you are uncomfortable talking about it?

182

Do you think that second honeymoons are a good idea? If you were going to take one, where would be the most romantic place you could go?

185

What would you do if the person you were so attracted to split up with your acquaintance—at least for the moment? How much do you care about whether or not you become an intrusive force in someone else's relationship? Has anyone ever moved in on a relationship of yours when you were having problems, and if so, how did you react?

200

Do you think you could be happy if you looked into the future and saw that you would never have a permanent mate or family?

206

What is the difference between being in love and being infatuated? Do you believe in "love at first sight"? Have you ever fallen in love largely because you so craved the intoxicating feelings of being in love? Do such feelings now seem more important or less important than they did when you were younger?

208

How much does your performance as a lover depend upon the partner you are with? Does it mean much to speak of someone as a "good" or "bad" lover, as though this is a personal quality that is independent of his or her partner? If so, how do you explain that two different people will sometimes have completely different experiences with a lover they have in common—for example, one might think the person is fabulous while the other thinks he or she is a complete dud?

216

If 20 years from now your child looks identical to the way your spouse looked in the bloom of youth, do you think parental and romantic feelings might get confused? What do you think it would be like to grow up having a parent who was an older version of yourself?

228

Do you and your partner make lifestyle choices specifically designed to set up or reduce day-to-day mutual dependencies? If so, why do you think you do so? How do you think your relationship would change if this dependence on each other became much greater or much less?

235

In what ways do you feel that parents should or should not hide sex and nudity from their young children? What about disagreements and conflicts in their relationship? How should a parent's openness about these things be different when kids are older or fully grown?

GREGORY STOCK is the author of THE BOOK OF QUESTIONS, which has been translated into 15 languages, THE KIDS' BOOK OF QUESTIONS, which is being used in schools around the country, and, most recently, THE BOOK OF QUESTIONS: BUSINESS, POLITICS AND ETHICS. He received a doctorate in biophysics from Johns Hopkins University in 1977, and has published numerous papers in biophysics and developmental biology. A Baker Scholar, he received an MBA from Harvard Business School in 1987.